The Food Lord

Seven Goes Grocery Shopping

Seven Ford & Antonio Ford

The Food Lord

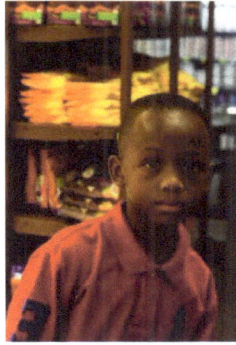

Seven Goes Grocery Shopping

Seven Ford
& Antonio Ford

Thank you....

I love to edutain! Hello, my name is Antonio Ford a.k.a. "The Food Lord." I like to thank God for providing me with the creative thought to keep bringing you the best food information yet. I want to thank William Crozier for believing in my vision and coming through for me.

I like to thank my children for their presence. I can't leave out Kat and Jeff for letting me borrow your son, Jordan Tenenbaum who brought my words to life with great photography. Thank you!

The incredible Curt Ashburn, thank you for making it possible for the world to know me!

Finally, I would like to thank my better half, Danielle Ford "Mrs. Food Lord."

Your skills make my work come to life. As my wife, you are my life. Thank you.

I cannot leave out the many supporters that purchased my previous works over the years. To my neighbor Antwaun Hawkins. You have no idea how our conversations motivated me to push forward with the new ideas!

The best is yet to come! Hope you enjoyed this super book as much as I did creating it.

FRESH! Antonio Ford

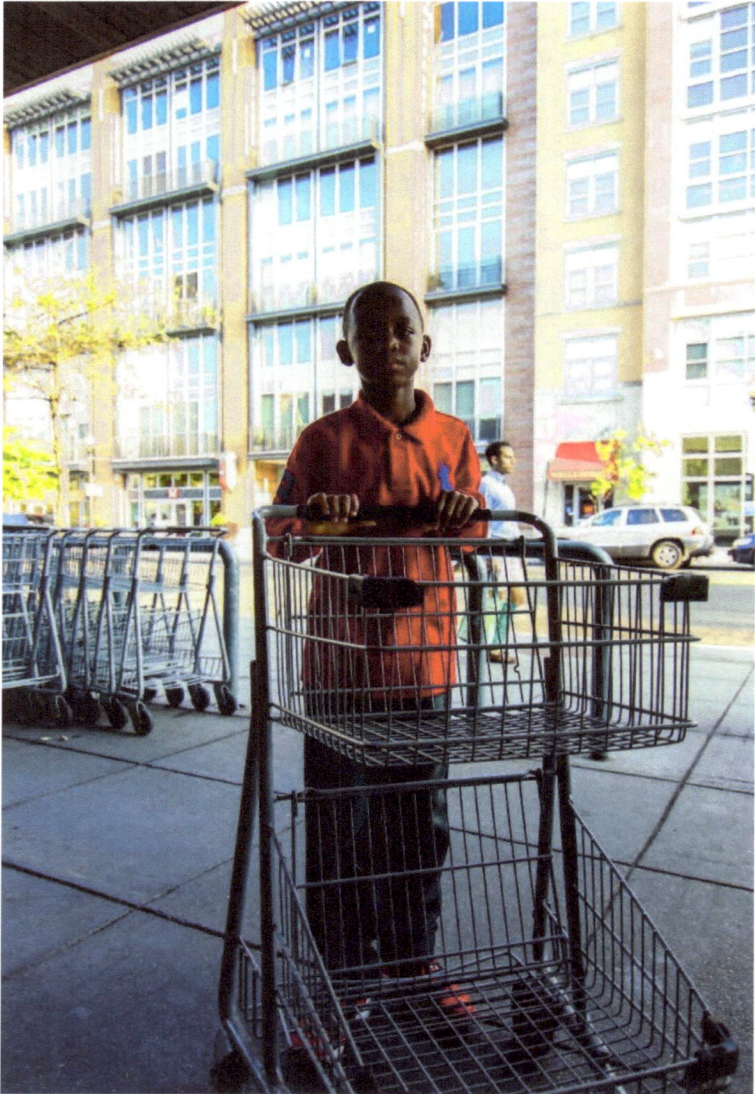

Hello, my name is Seven Ford. Would you like to go grocery shopping with me?

We must make a grocery list first….

Seven's Grocery List

- ✓ Raspberries
- ✓ Natural Cereal
- ✓ Water
- ✓ Cashew Milk
- ✓ Orange Juice (Not from Concentrate)
- ✓ Peas
- ✓ Brussel Sprouts

Let's see… When my Mom takes me grocery shopping with her, she normally goes to the produce section first. This is the produce section. It is my favorite place because it has so many yummy foods that are so good for you.

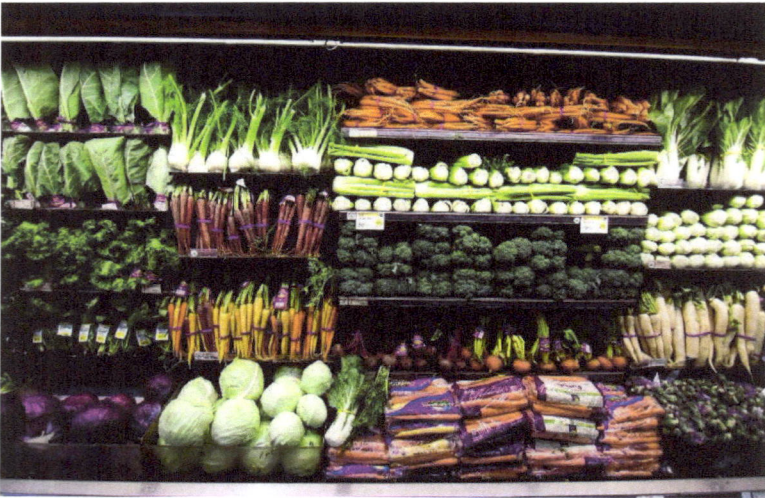

Look at all the colorful fruits, cherries, apples, and
pomegranates … Here, are the raspberries.

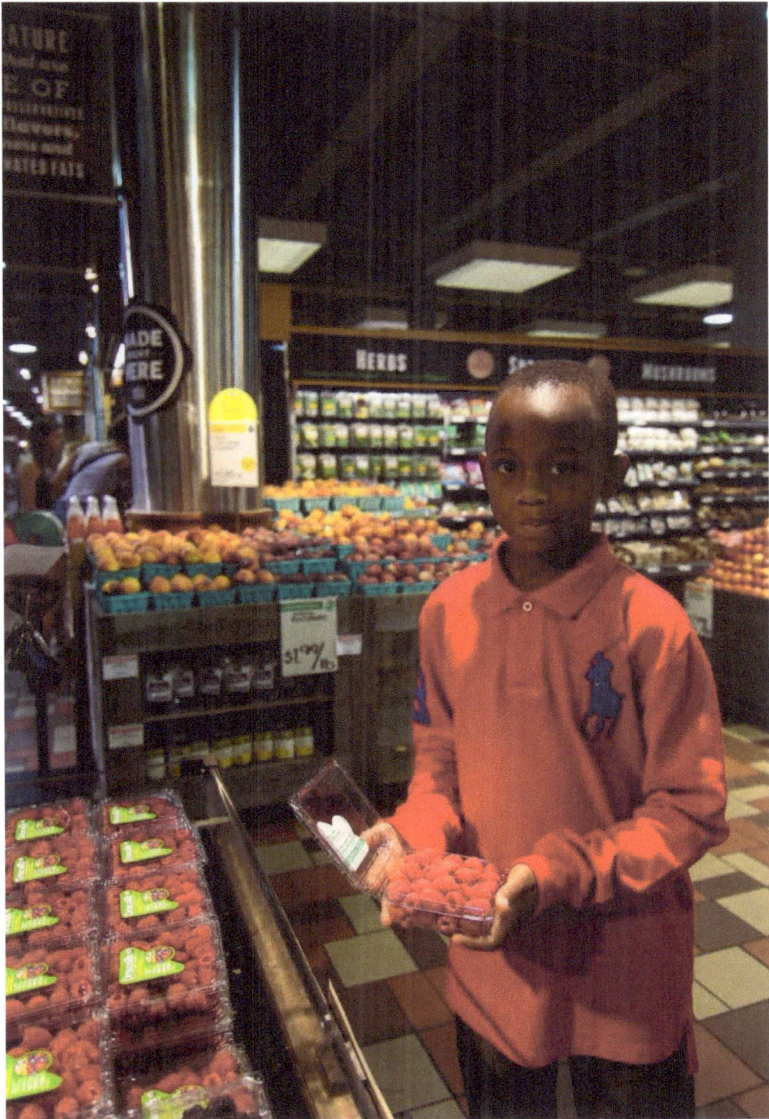

Next, the Brussel sprouts and peas.

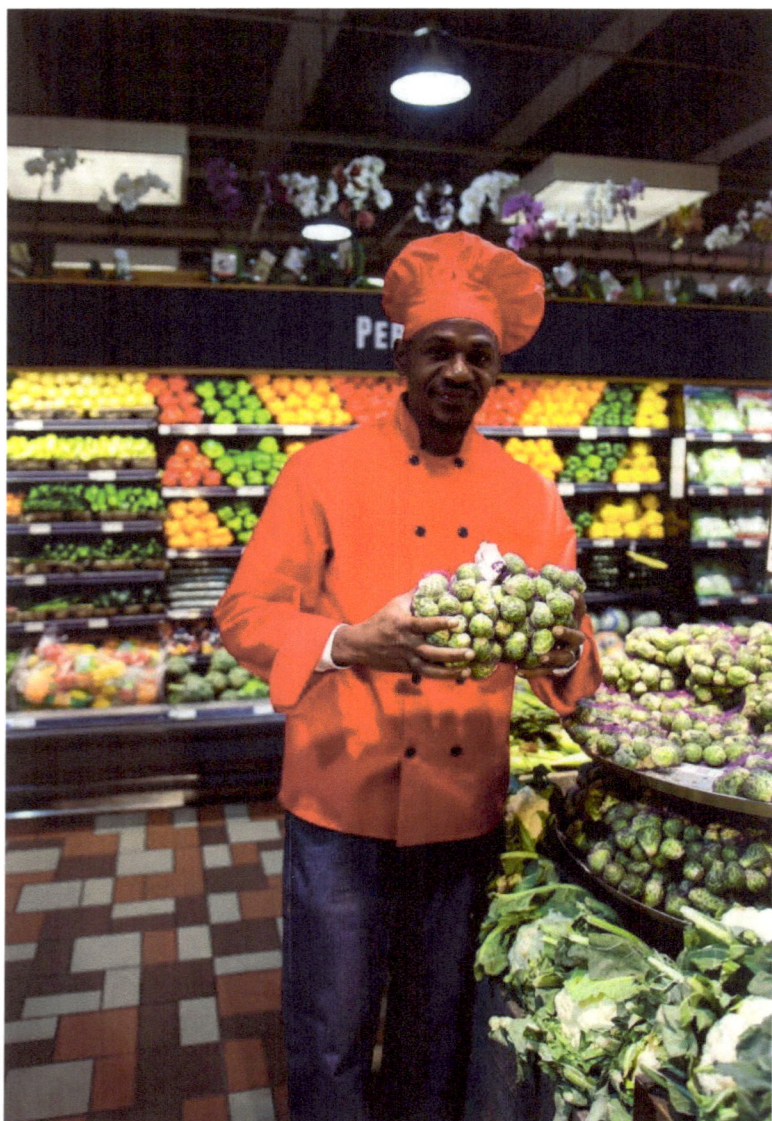

These are Brussel Sprouts. My dad calls them
"Superfoods." I like to eat them raw or cooked.

My dad says they are a great source of protein. The
next time you go to the grocery store, pick up a
handful.

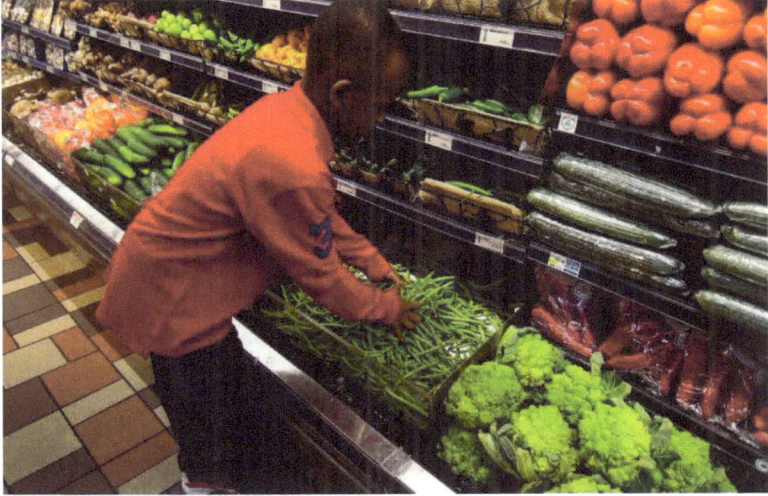

I think most kids love sting beans. They are yummy and packed with proteins and other essential nutrients for growing children like us.

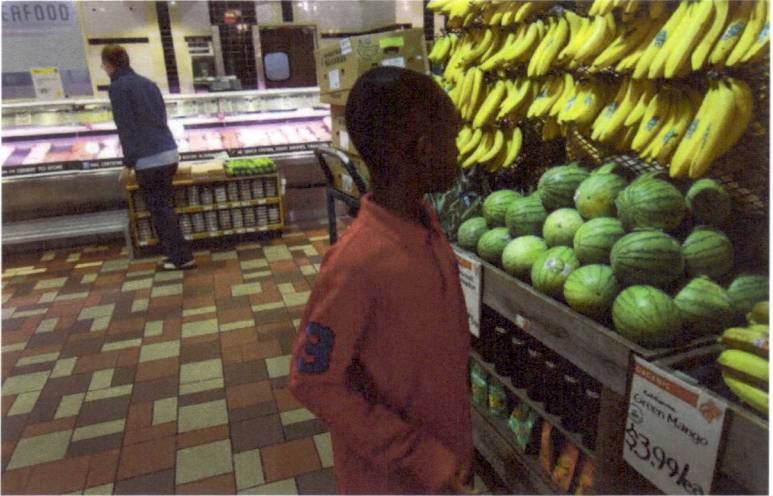

When you see fruits that are GMO, don't stop to buy them. GMO foods come with NO seeds and promote health defects.

Let's go to the cereal aisle. I never eat the sugary cereals. They are mostly artificial and loaded with sugar or high fructose corn syrup which is bad for the immune system. I love Honey'd Corn Flakes. Let's put these into the cart.

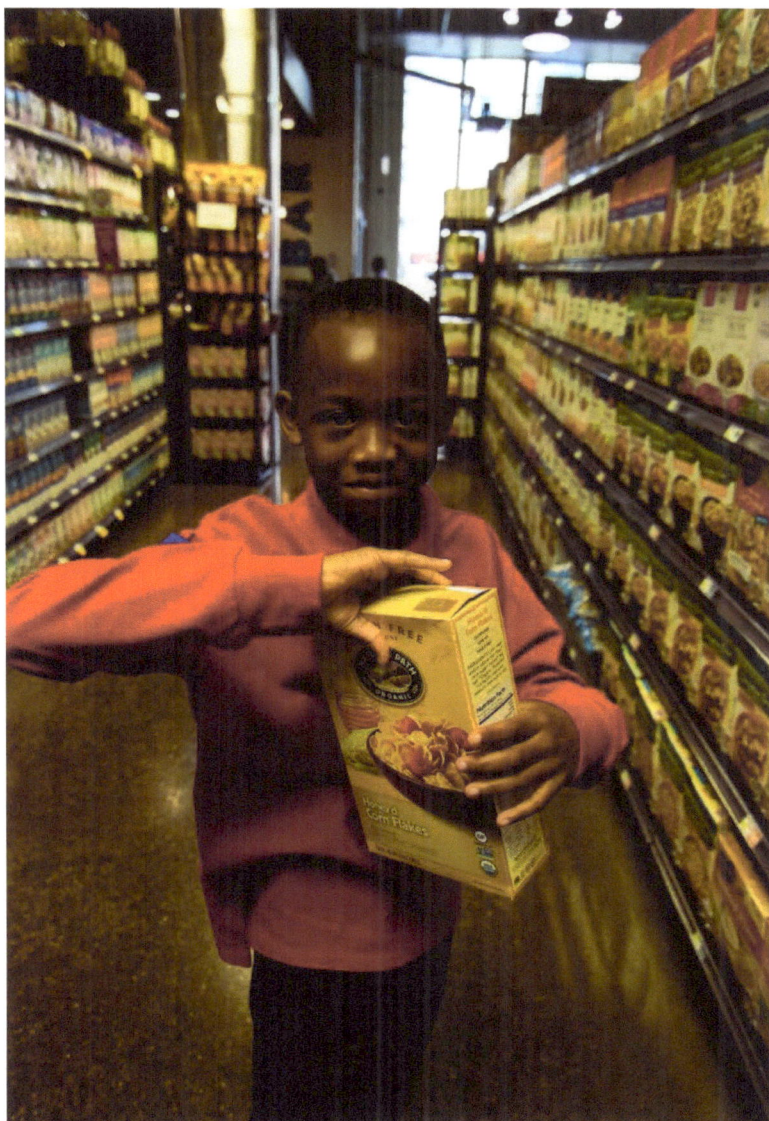

What else am I missing from my list?

I need to find the Cashew Milk... Wait, here it is.

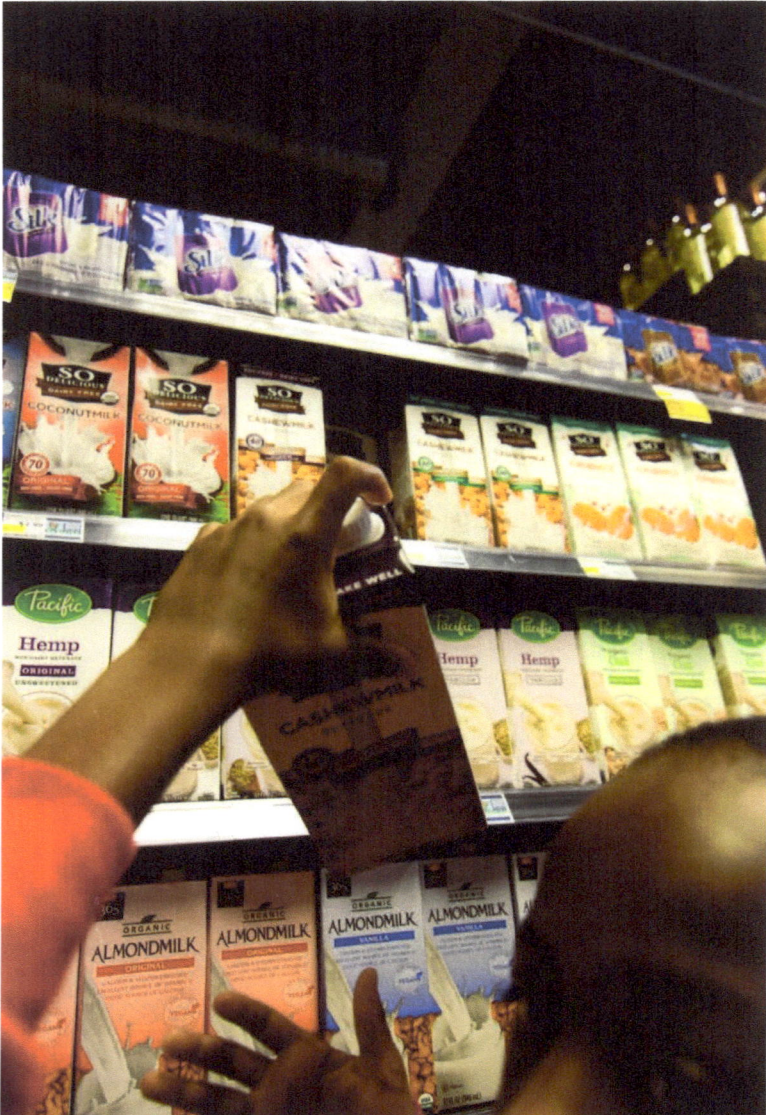

One of the biggest myths about milk is that cow's milk is good for you, but cow's milk leaves cholesterol in your body.

I used to drink soymilk but, my dad taught me that soymilk isn't good for your body either. It's too rich for the body and raises the estrogen levels in both men and women.

That's not good for growing boys' and girls' growth and development.

Now, I drink cashew milk. Cashews are rich in protein which is great for growing bones. It tastes better than cow's milk and it comes in chocolate too!

Your milk should read, "NON-GMO" too!

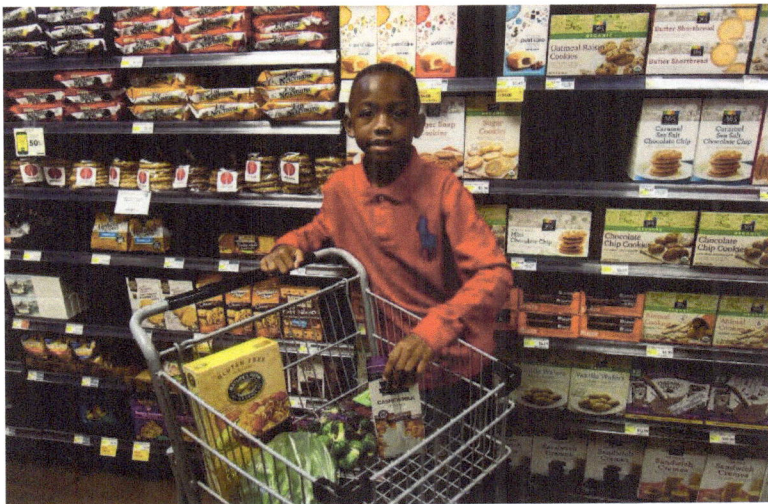

This is my first time picking out the items on my own at the grocery store. I am so excited to pick out healthy food to eat.

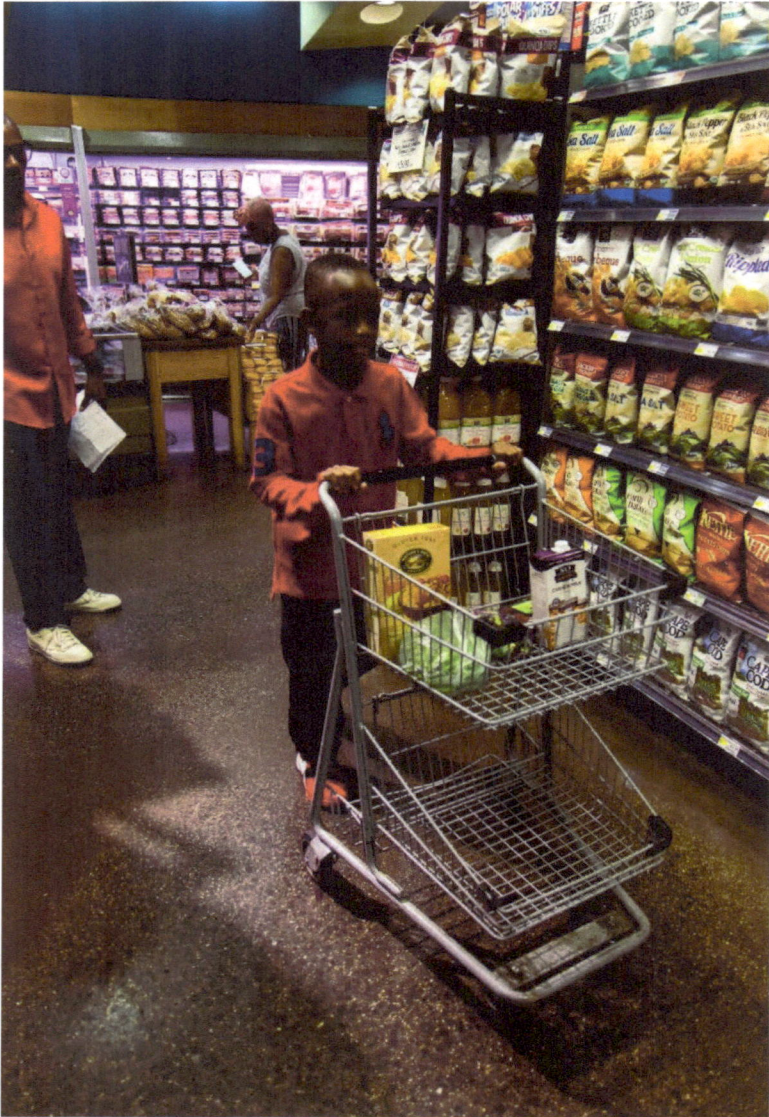

In the beverage aisle, you will find all kinds of juices mostly from concentrate. Some juices have 12% juice, some 10% juice, but they are all from concentrate.

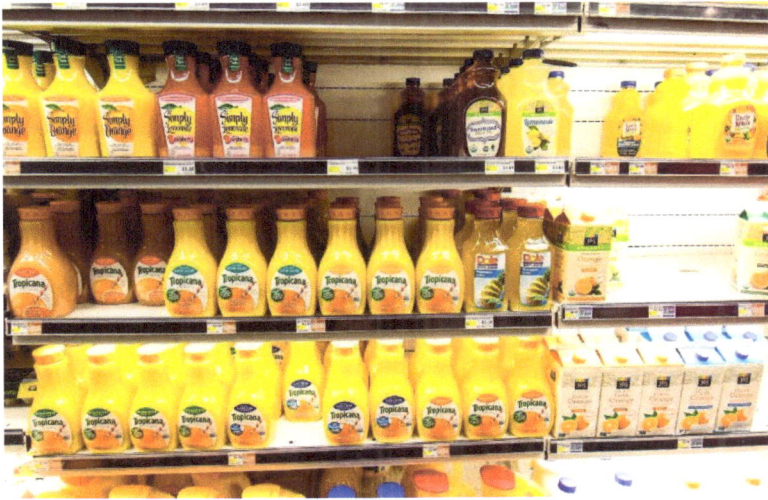

My dad says that drinking juices from concentrate is bad for you. They eventually cause diabetes. He recommends that everyone drink juices that say "NEVER" or "NOT FROM CONCENTRATE" are best for our bodies.

My juice is not from concentrate and is always 100% juice. It also has a NON-GMO label on it too!

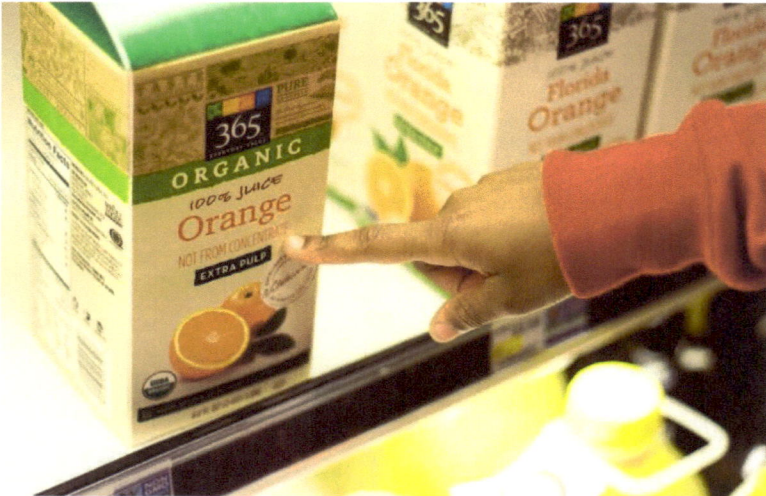

Water! I love drinking water. In fact, I drink more water than anything. Do you drink water? Let me encourage you to drink at least four 8oz. cups per day. Another great thing that I like to do is put a few berries into my water to infuse it.

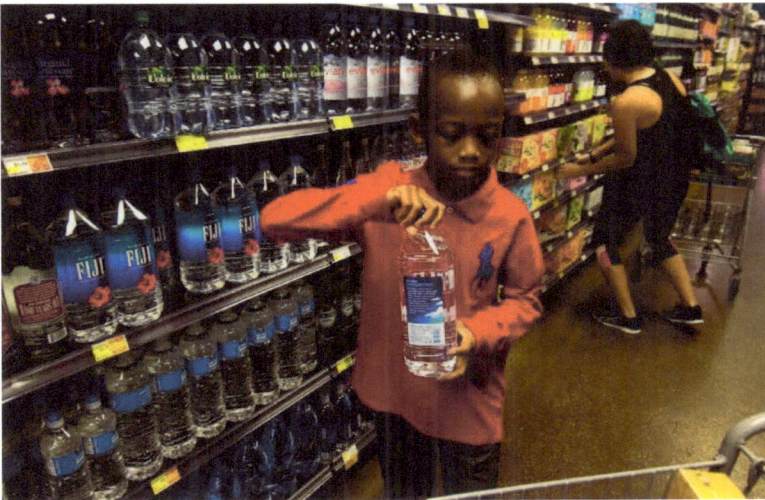

I think that I have everything that I need and now I can go to the register and get checked out.

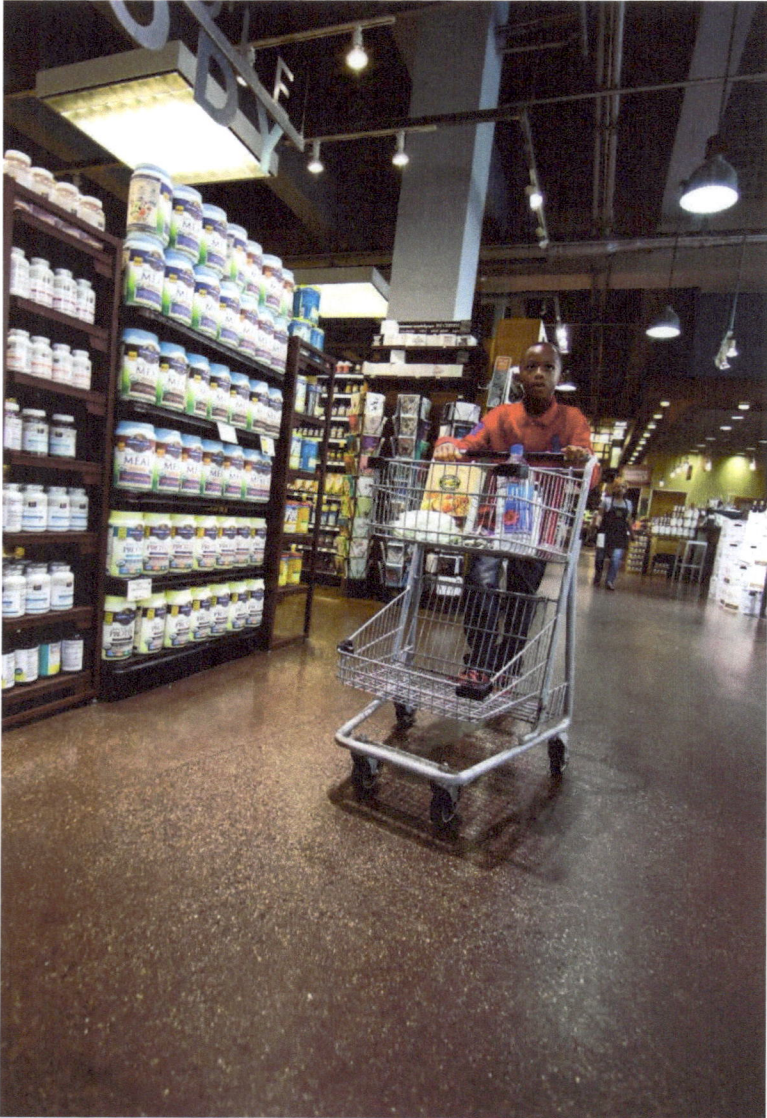

Cashier: Hello there! What is your name? Where is your Mom or Dad?

Seven: My name is Seven and my dad is right over there. He allowed me to grocery shop on my own while he watched me.

Cashier: Well, put your items on the conveyer belt and I will take care of you.

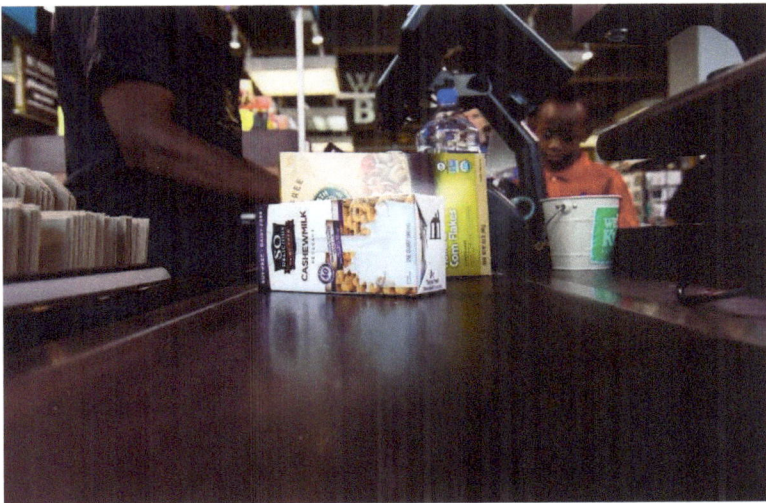

Cashier: OK Seven, your total today is $18.07

Seven: Here is a $20.00-dollar bill

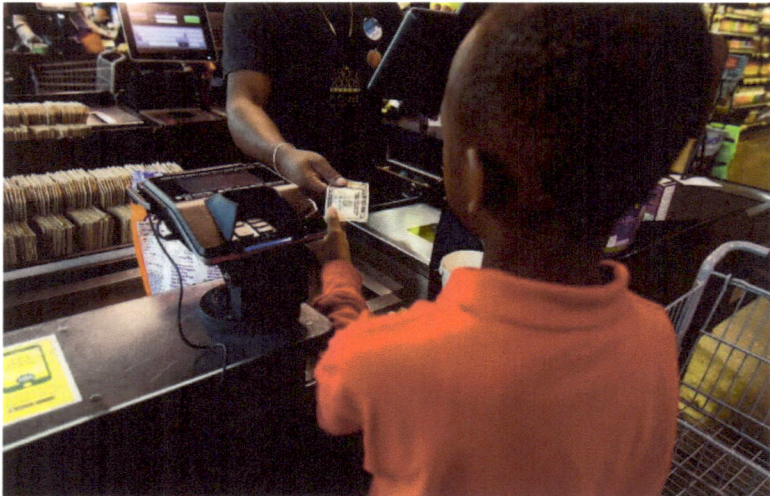

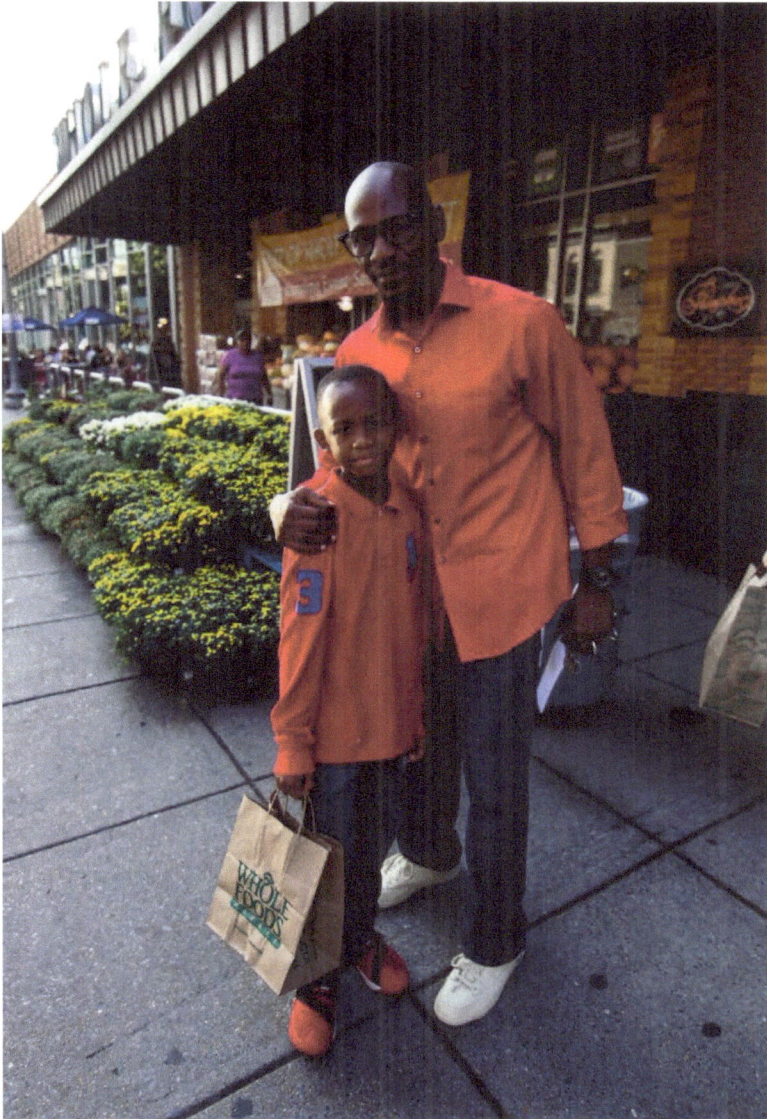

Dad, I did it! I did it! I went grocery shopping on my own! I had so much fun today. I hope that you did too. Remember to eat for health and keep in mind it's one bite at a time.

Catch you later… Fresh!
Seven Ford

The End

www.ingramcontent.com/pod-product-compliance
Lightning Source LLC
Chambersburg PA
CBHW041227270326
41934CB00001B/30